This Page is Intentionally Left Blank

# Table of Contents

# A Collage of Happiness

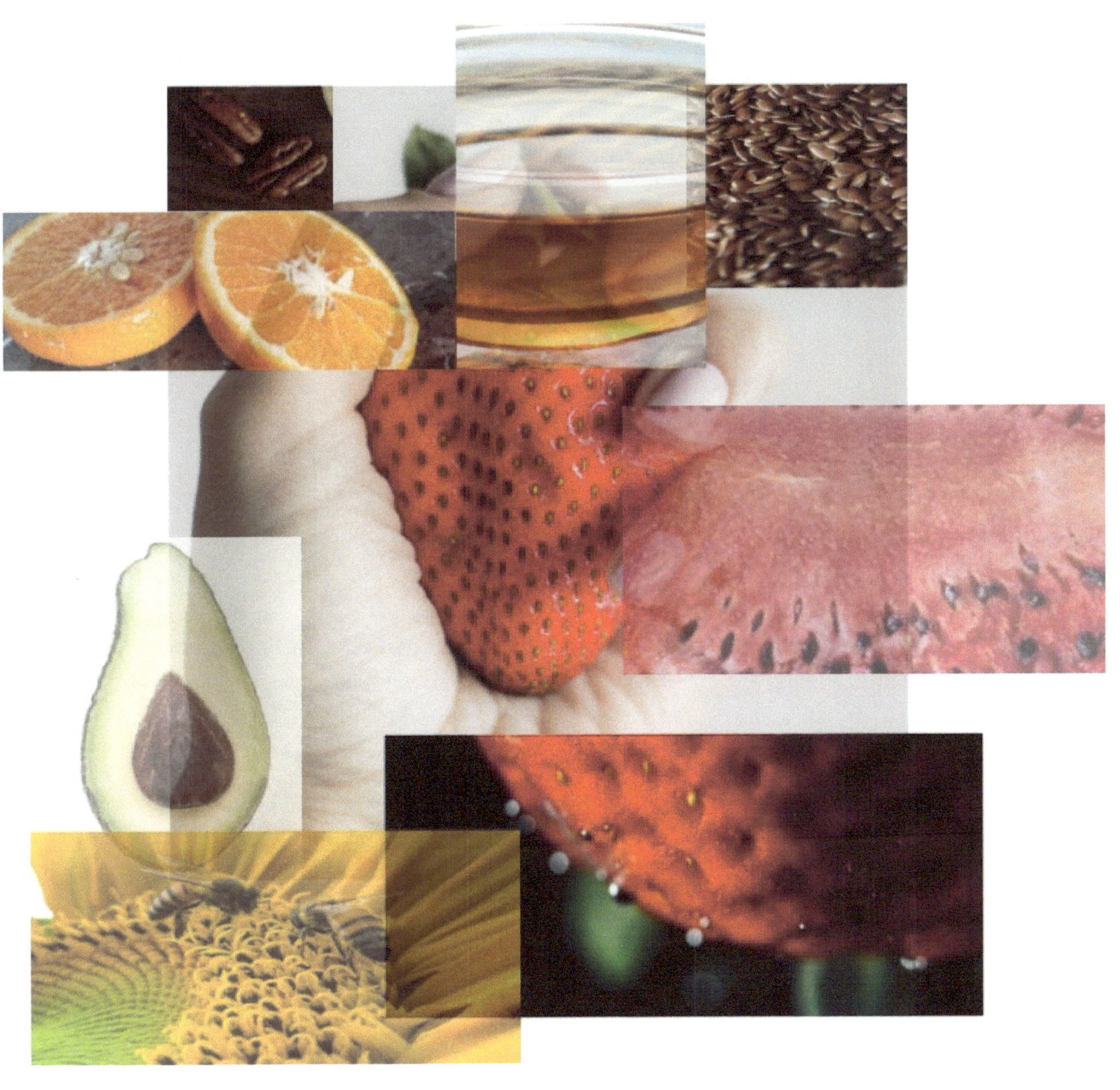

# The Seven Best Nutritious Smoothie Recipes Ever: Costs Less, Tastes Great and Lose Weight.

## Introduction

Smoothies are one of the easiest and most convenient ways to stay on track with weight loss goals while treating yourself to something that's both delicious and nutritious. Blend one up for breakfast, to take with you to work for a mid-morning pick-me-up, or enjoy after a workout.

The basis for your smoothie should typically be plain yogurt for protein, nuts or seeds for fat and more protein, a small serving of fruit for carbs (and because it will taste better with a little sweetness), and perhaps a bit of something green for extra nutrition. You can also include good-for-you additions like frozen tart cranberries, flaxseed or avocado.

To make a smoothie, just take out the blender and add in the nuts or seeds first. If they're whole, give a quick blend on the grind setting. Next add in frozen fruit or veggie such as spinach. You can skip adding ice if you put in a frozen ingredient or two. If not using frozen produce, add some ice if you like. Next add in fresh fruit. Top with yogurt and fill to your desired height with a liquid like soymilk, regular milk, or even water. Blend thoroughly, pour into a glass and enjoy. Nothing cooler than a beautifully made smoothie.

## Rethinking Meals to Facilitate Weight Loss in a Jiffy

Sometimes, being successful about weight loss requires us to rethink the social attitudes and expectations about food that have been ingrained in us. One strategy for losing weight more easily is changing your view of meals, and how much or what type of food is eaten at a particular time of day.

In American society, it is customary to eat three meals a day, and some people snack as well. Breakfast can vary depending on personal preference, ranging from something small like a bagel on the run, to a sit-down morning meal with representation from all four food groups. Lunch might consist of a sandwich or mid-sized meal such as a salad with protein, and crackers or a piece of bread. Dinner typically is the biggest meal of all.

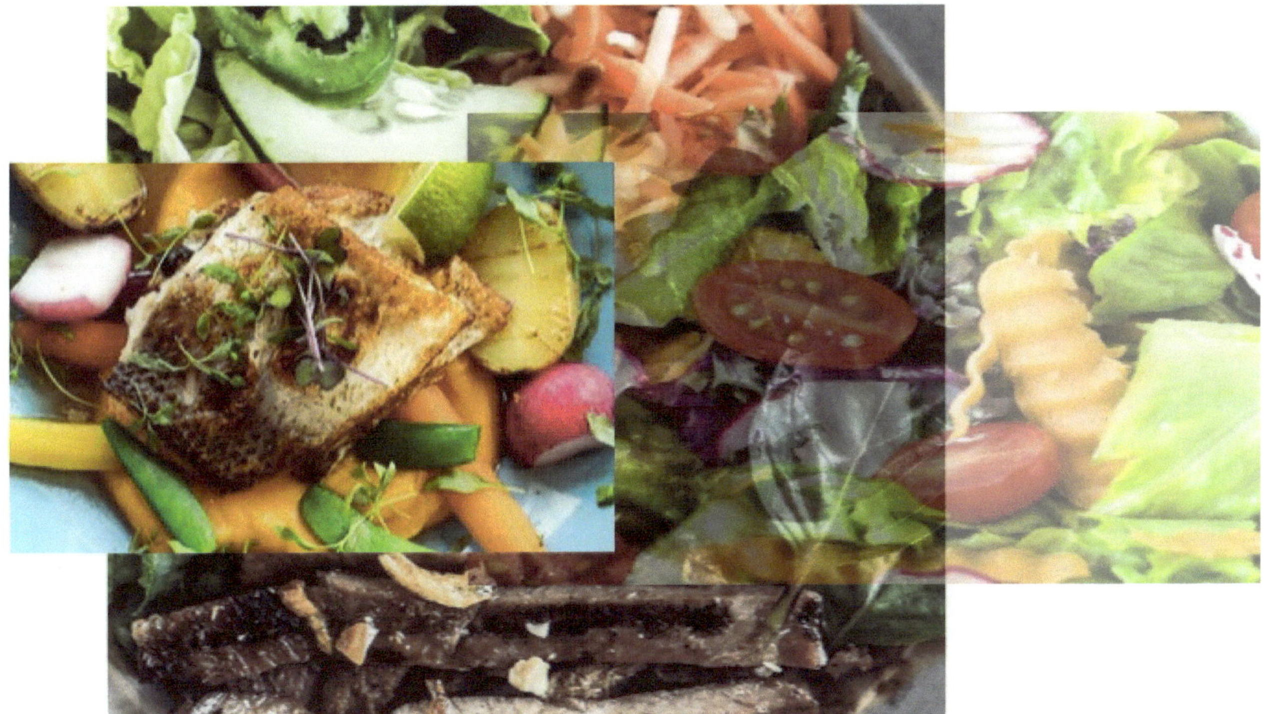

*Protein Salads*

Some people swear by a top-heavy daily meal schedule that has us eating the most food at breakfast, followed by a mid-sized lunch and light dinner. This may make sense because it has us consuming the bulk of our calories first, which gives us a full day of activity to burn off the energy. It also has the digestive system bearing most of its work load during waking hours when we're out and about, with time to rest while we're asleep.

Other people opt for the "intermittent fasting" method of losing weight. This means that they are actually skipping breakfast altogether, staying in overnight fasting mode from the evening hours to the next morning, past the usual time that they might typically eat breakfast.

The number of hours that people choose to intermittently fast really depends on personal preference. Some abstain from eating for about 16 hours, starting after dinner and continuing to the next day. Others fast for 12 hours and then indulge in a nutritious, mid-morning meal. Improved brain health, detox benefits, reduced inflammation and improved weight loss are 4 reasons why intermittent fasting may prove beneficial if you're trying to shed pounds and get healthy (15).

Another way to think differently about meals is to shake preconceived notions about what foods are appropriate for the time of day and meal. We think of cereal with milk, muffins or bagels as breakfast foods. But with so many people limiting their intake of carbs, especially white flour and sugary foods, in an effort to lose weight and avoid chronic illness, this has us rethinking what to have for the first meal of the day.

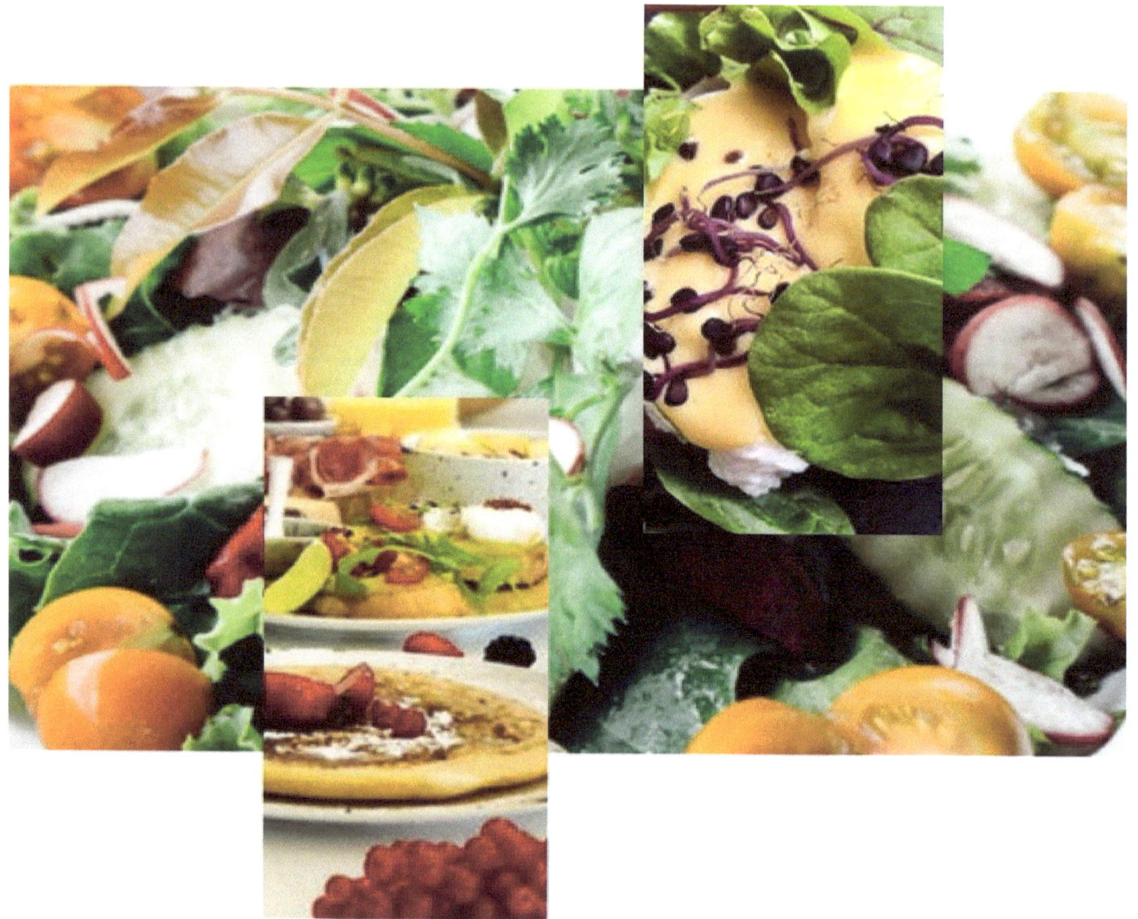

## Breakfast Salads

As more people branch out, trying new ways of eating such as the ketogenic diet, it's becoming more commonplace to eat breakfasts that seem more like lunch or even dinner. Lean protein such as turkey, cooked with egg whites, served with half a sweet potato and a cup of dressed greens, could be what breakfast looks like to increasingly health-conscious eaters who are looking for ways to vary their meals and find what works to help them shed fat and unwanted pounds.

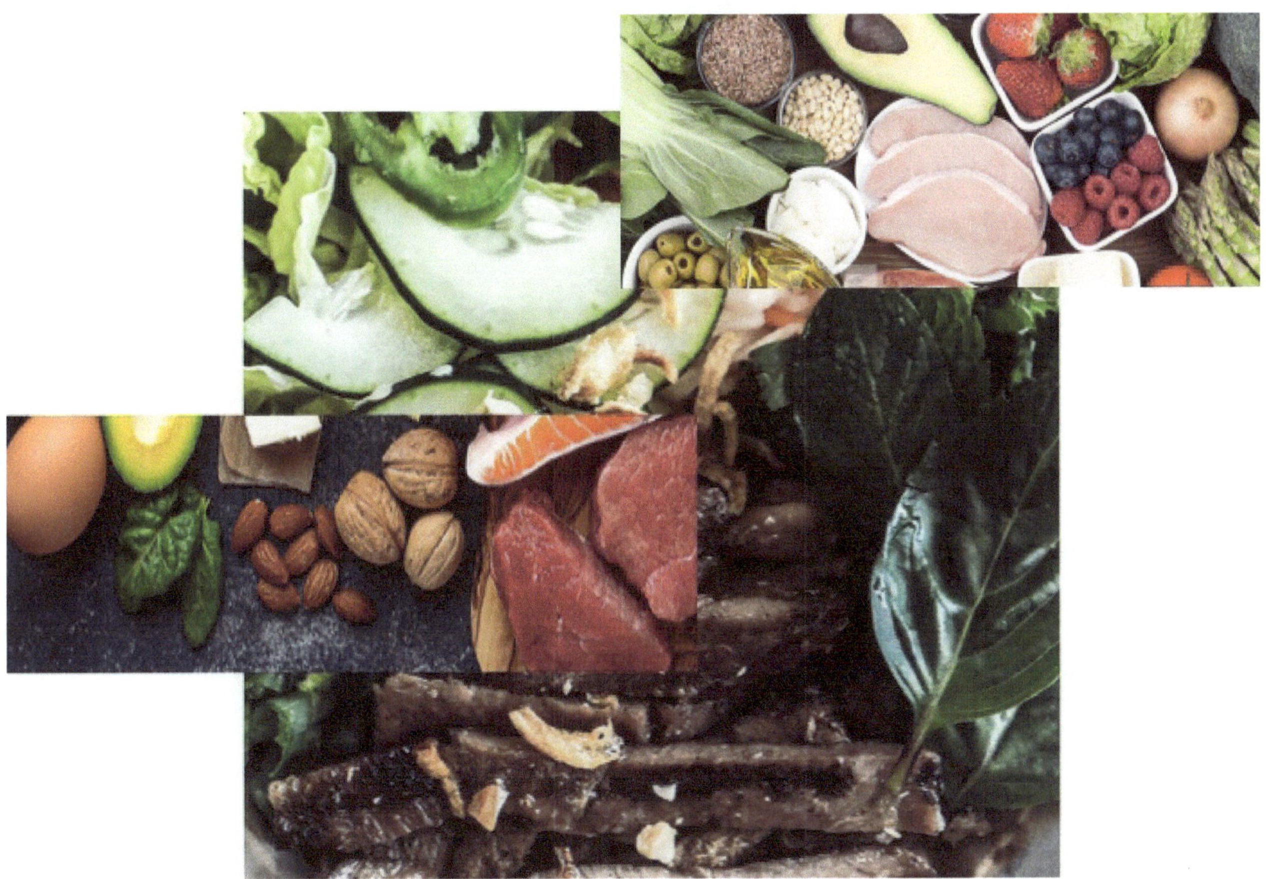



The important thing about changing the way you view meals is to figure out what works for you. In order to do that, keep an open mind, and be willing to try different things.

If you aren't a person who feels hungry first thing in the morning, then make lunch your big meal of the day. If your work hours leave you with little time to sit down for lunch, then make sure to have plenty of small, healthy snack breaks throughout your busy day.

# Reducing Calories Without Compromising Nutrition or Sacrificing Taste.

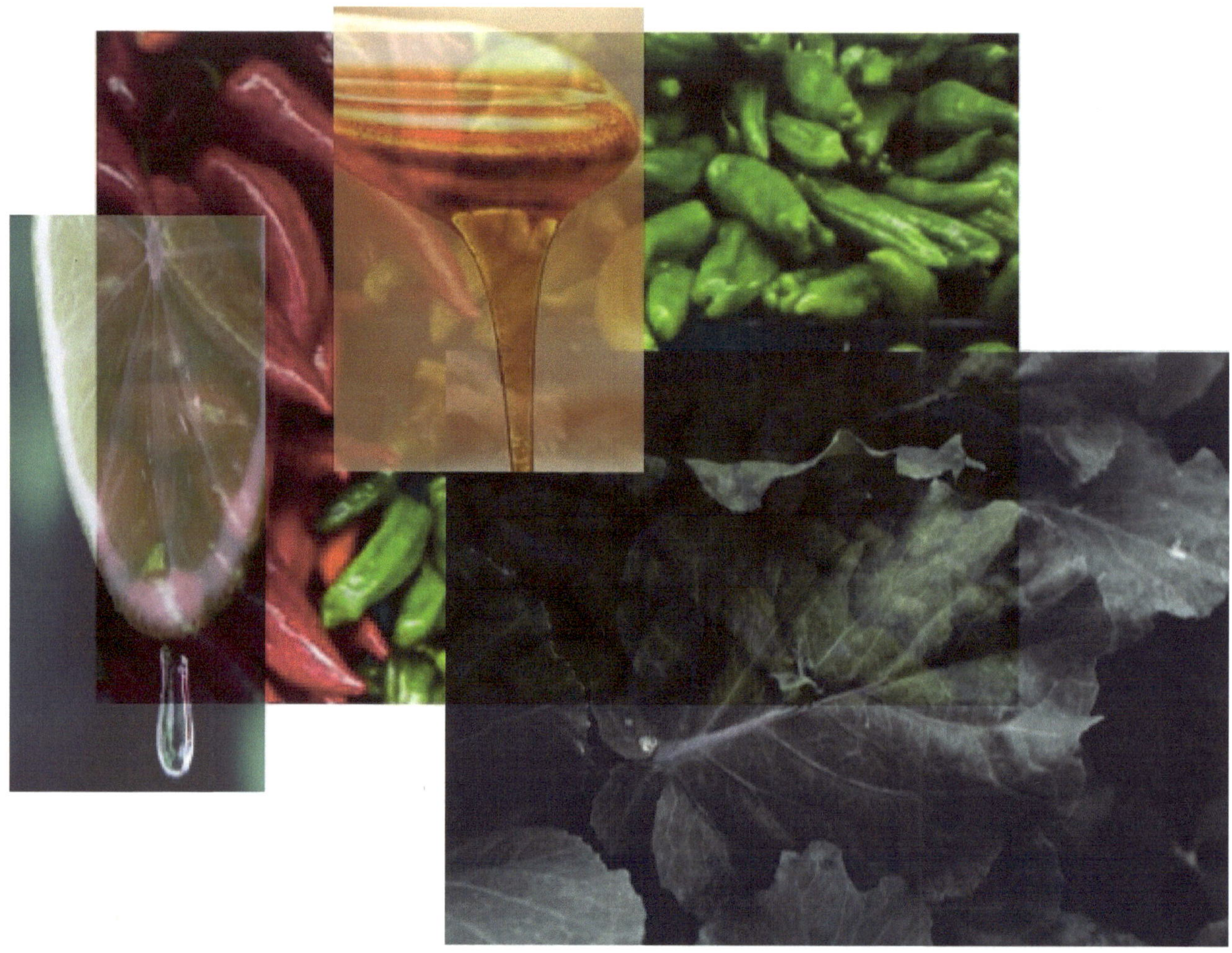

*Let's Talk About Taste*

Looking for a simple nutritional plan to follow so you can lose weight? Typically, the reason why we gain weight in the first place is because we are consuming more calories than we're burning off in our daily activities. So, we can either increase the amount of exercise we do each day in order to expend more energy, or we can eat less... or some combo of both.

In addition to balancing intake and burning off of calories (which are really just energy units), we should also consider the type and quality of foods we eat on a regular basis.

Traditional nutritional advice maintains that a balanced diet consist of about 50% carbs, with the other half of our daily calorie intake made up of about 20% protein and 30% fat, give or take. However, those who have embarked on the ketogenic way of eating are doing completely different nutritional numbers - the bulk of which are comprised of fats, with extremely low carb counts.

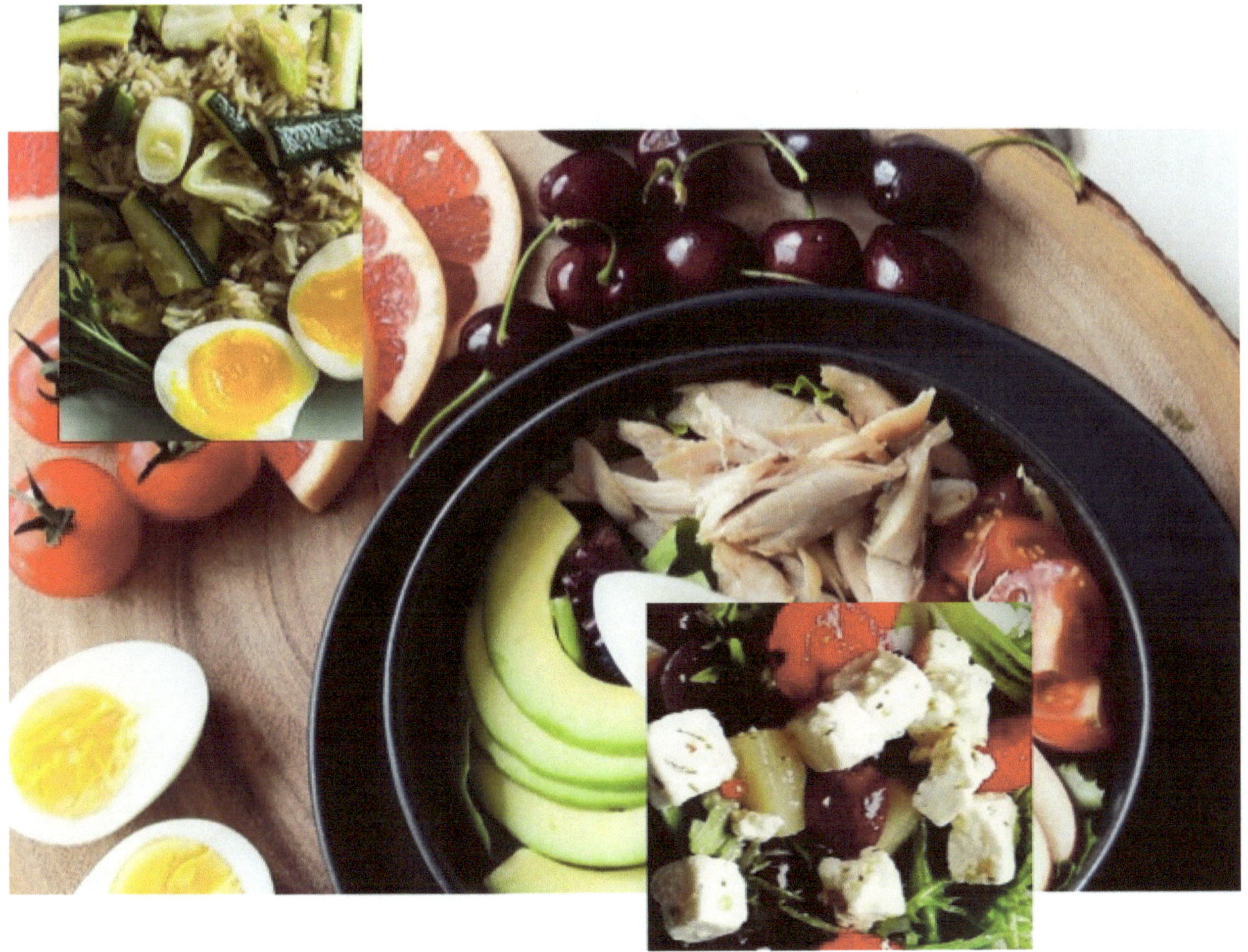



If you are not into carb-counting and high fat foods don't sit well in your stomach, then a low-carb diet may not be right for you. In that case, it's a smart idea to take the traditional 50% carbs approach, but do it in a healthy way. Switch from white flour to whole grain products such as pasta and bread. Choose brands of bread that do not contain added sugar, and if you're not sure about amounts then check and compare total number of carbs per serving for different brands.

Another way to fill up on good carbs is to consider your vegetable intake as part of your total carbs for the day. So, if you eat three baby carrots, a slice of wheat bread and some nut butter for lunch, then you must think of the carrots as counting toward your total carb load. In other words, refrain from eating that second slice of bread.

People who eat half a sandwich with a side salad are already doing this; they just maybe are not thinking of it in terms of being a numbers game, but that's what they've been trained to do. Another example of this is if, as a dieter, you'd have a cup of vegetable soup with half a sandwich on whole grain bread. You may think of this as a "dieting strategy" but it's actually a better way to eat that we are not used to with our American tendency toward too-large portions and empty-calorie foods.

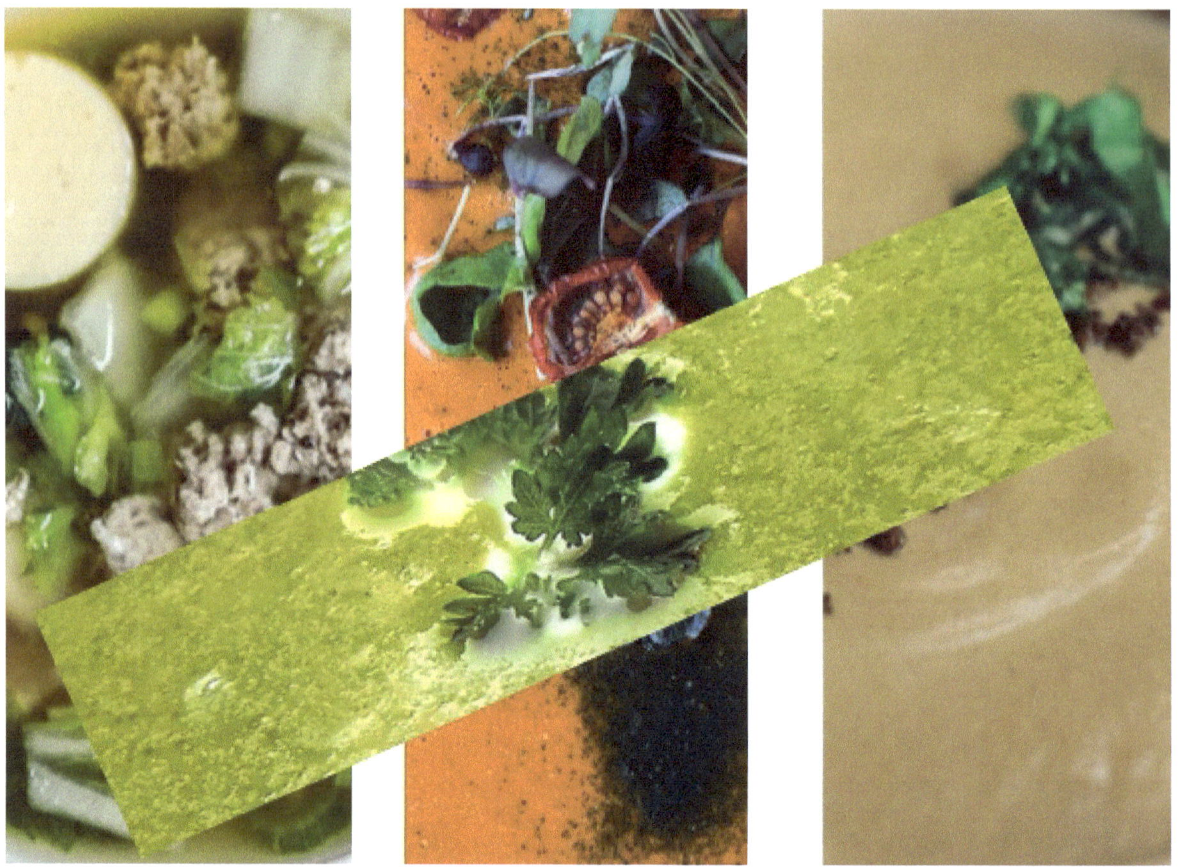



Here's a tip for limiting the effects of sugar while still enjoying the occasional dessert. When you do splurge on a sweet treat, pair it with fiber to give your pancreas and liver a break. For example, a sweetened muffin that's made from whole grain and contains nuts, seeds and dried fruits will digest more slowly thanks to the fiber. But a processed, empty-calorie muffin made from enriched white flour sends high amounts of sugar straight to the liver and blood stream. This makes your organs work extra hard and contributes to chronic disease such as diabetes and heart trouble, over the long term.

More tips for upping the flavor factor while making healthy eating choices:

Use herbs, aromatics, healthy oils, and spices to season your lean meats. A baked chicken breast seems boring, but how satisfying would that lean meat be if cooked with olive oil, Balsamic vinegar, garlic, onions and peppers? It's really all about artful food combinations, and there is usually science behind which foods taste best together. For example, vinegar helps to break down the protein and fat that you consume, as well as enhances absorption of vitamins and minerals from your vegetables.

# The Trick is to Trick Yourself into Being Full

Let's Ask ourselves these questions for a start:

Are you hungry all of the time? Are you trying to lose weight, but you just can't seem to do it because of constant hunger?

Do you have trouble keeping the weight off because you're consumed (no pun intended) with cravings for all the wrong foods that raise your blood sugar, increase body fat and pack on the pounds?

Do you find that small portions just aren't satisfying and you end up refilling your plate for seconds and even thirds?

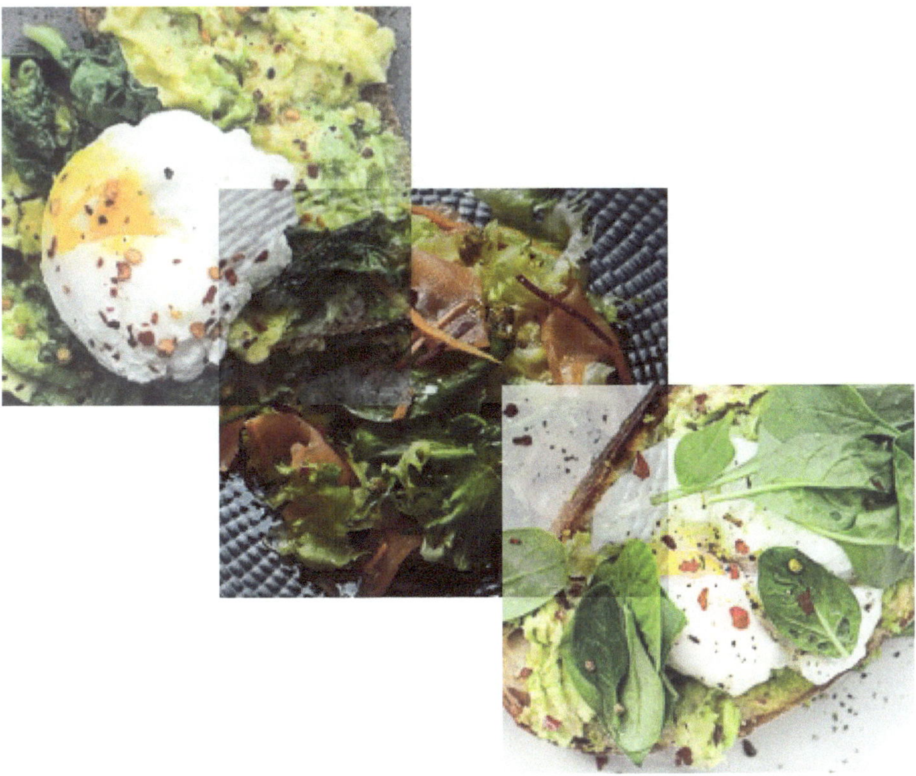

*Eating in small Portions*
The ideas offered below are not really tricks after all… but they are a new way of thinking which can help you eat less often and smaller portions.

Sometimes hunger is more of psychological thing than a physiological one. So, if we really want to lessen the amount and increase the quality of the food that we put into our bodies, then one of the first big steps we can take is to change our thoughts and feelings around being hungry.

Is there a way to tell when you're legitimately hungry, versus having a craving, or wanting to fill our bellies for emotional reasons?

Can we "trick" ourselves into feeling less hungry?

One confirmative way to know if it's legitimate hunger versus emotional eating or eating to pass the time, is to figure out when was your last nutritious meal. Most people need to refuel their bodies with good, nutritious foods about every 4 hours. Some may need a small snack sooner than that.

This sounds simple to abide by... to eat a meal very few hours. But if it was so easy to do, then why are so many of us hooked on fattening snacks, loading up on donuts, chips, and other bad-for-you foods?

Suppose your lunch consisted of a scoop of tuna, a slice of rye bread, carrot sticks, and a glass of lemon water. That was at noon, and now it's 3 p.m. You want something satisfying. Are you truly hungry? Of course, whether your body truly needs to refuel depends on how large you are, how big the scoop of tuna was, and how many calories you burned between then and now.

Maybe the 3 hours between lunch and now were especially stressful. If that's the case, your body may be crying out for something. You burned calories and your cortisol levels are high due to the stressful situation.

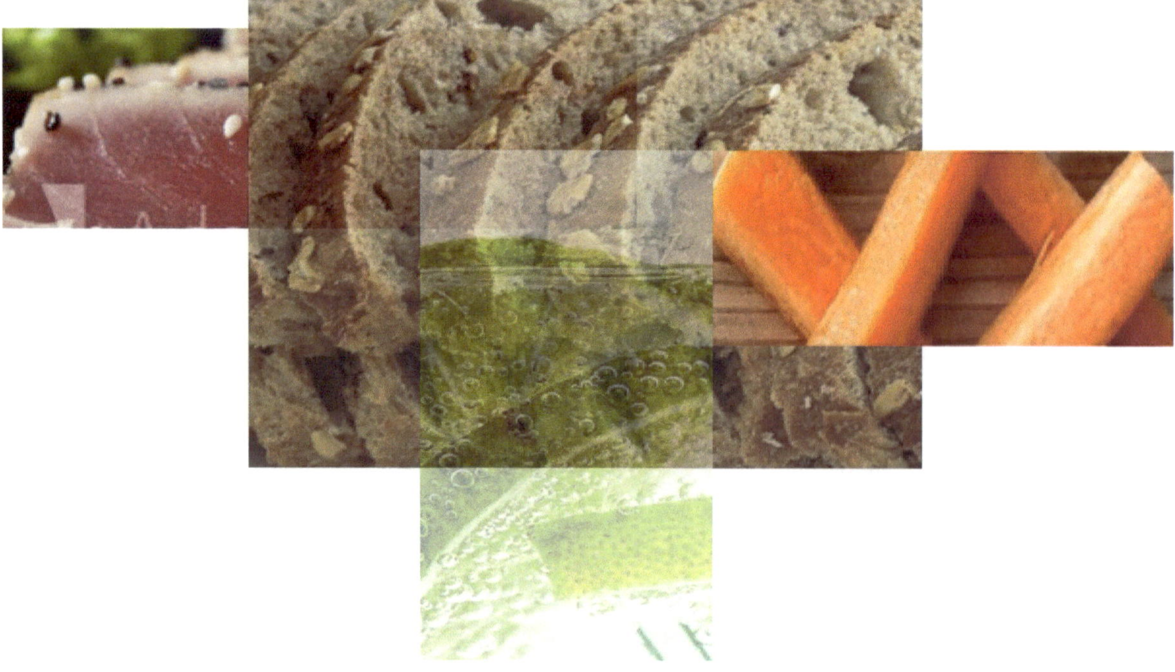

*The Tuna-Carrots-Lemon water Lunch*

Do you really need that sugary snack? Or is your brain asking for some feel-good serotonin? Protein will settle the nerves and deliver nourishment to the muscles and brain. So, reach for a handful of nuts. Chew them slowly and mindfully. How about a slice or two of fruit? Now you've given your body what it really needs, without heading into unhealthy snack territory.

Another reason you might have a hungry feeling, or a wild craving, is yeast overgrowth. Every being has yeast living in their body, so some amount of it is normal. But yeast can get out of control in our digestive tract after a course of antibiotics, or if we over-indulge in alcohol or eat lots of sugary foods.

If you're feeling low and like you need a sweet pick-me-up, it could be the yeast beasts in your digestive system. Try adding coconut oil to your diet. A spoonful of this healthy fat taken in the morning, afternoon and evening can be very satisfying. Coconut oil curbs hunger, kills yeast and is good for the body in many other ways.

Know what else can contribute to hunger? Not chewing your food completely when eating. People who eat too fast without taking time to chew tend not to absorb all of the nutrition from their food.

It cannot be over emphasized that, if you want to feel hungry less often, chew your food thoroughly. It's said that we should chew each mouthful of food at least 30 times if we want to promote healthy digestion. Plus, when we chew thoroughly, we give our bodies time to digest, and our brains get the message that we're full. Rushing through meals doesn't give our brain the signal to know that we're satisfied and have had our fill of needed nutrition.

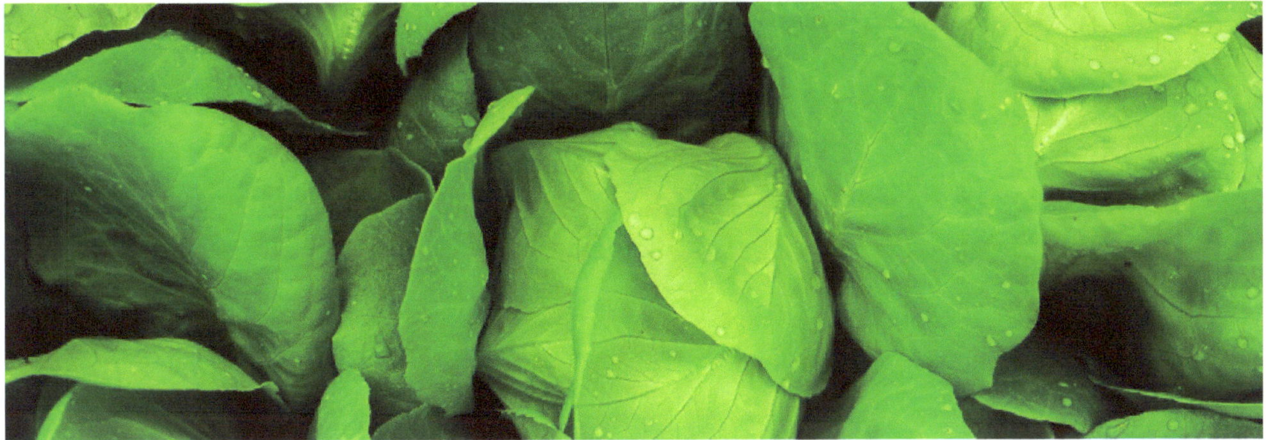

*Spinach*

Did you know that digestion begins in the mouth? As we chew, enzymes in our saliva begin to break down the food we eat. Our teeth masticate the food into tiny pieces, and finally, into a paste that we then swallow. This self-made pate contains all the nutrition that our body needs to process to stay healthy.

Another reason why it's important to chew is that when you gulp down large chunks of food, your stomach must work harder to process it. Parts of your meal may go undigested, become stuck in, and irritate the lining of your stomach. If you eat this way all the time, it can result in an inflamed stomach and intestinal lining.

After being inflamed for a while, your stomach can develop tears and perforations. These tears cause protein from your food to enters your blood stream. When protein molecules enter the blood, your body sends out antibodies to fight the perceived attacker or foreign substance. You develop allergy-like symptoms and chronic inflammation.

So, think about that the next time you're wolfing down dinner. Your body will be a lot better off if you salivate and chew your food completely. And when your nutritional needs are met, you won't feel quite as hungry so soon.

Other ways to help your mind and body to not feel hungry:

Stretch to reduce stress. Stress sends a signal to our brain that it wants something. It's craving that high, that mellow feeling that a big meal or a sugary snack can provide. This is, believe it or not, an addiction! However, you needn't be a slave to sugar. Doing yoga and other light stretches at various points of your day can rid your body of the stress chemicals that make you feel hungry.

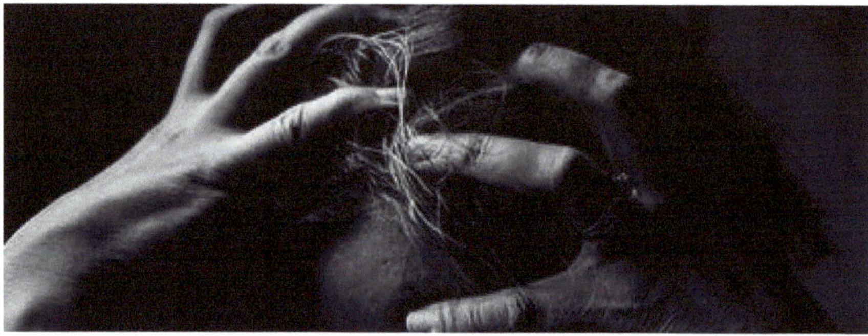

*Life can Be Stressful Sometimes*

Next time you feel stressed-out hungry, stop and do a few deep stretches. Then, assess your hunger to see if you're still as ravenous as you think you are. Instead of having that slice of cake, you may find yourself satisfied with just a small snack, like hummus and a few pieces of celery.

# Some Fruit and Vegetable Insights

We all have our own ideas on what we considered healthy food alternatives based on past experiences, what we may have eating, seen or read about. One "best" food from a region of the world may be a taboo in another. S the saying goes, "beauty is always in the eye of the beholder". Improving our nutritional health and food intakes may be focused solely on nutrient laden foods. However, these may not turn out to be best based on calorie intakes, sugars, allergies and taste.

As far as smoothies go it is about chemistry. The premise of this book is to group together ingredients even though may not at first look interesting but turns out great, tasty and very health to the point of proving the requited vitamins and minerals to sustain a person for some time. Feeling full for a while is the key.

Take for example Kale

Kale (11) at first look is bad tasting but in combination with other nutritious ingredients as we will see later provides and a very filling option, for a time in its sustaining ability. Thereby indirectly supporting positive weight correction.

Kale (mg/100 g fresh weight)

      Ascorbic acid - 105

      Thiamine - 0.10

      Riboflavin - 0.26

      Nicothiniacid - 2.10

      Folacid – 0.19

      $\alpha$-Tocopherol [Vitamin E] - 1.7

      $\beta$-Carotene - 5.2


Another example:

Spinach (mg/100 g fresh weight)

      Ascorbic acid - 51

      Thiamine - 0.10

      Riboflavin - 0.20

      Nicothiniacid – 0.6

      Folacid – 0.15

      $\alpha$-Tocopherol [Vitamin E] - 1.3

      $\beta$-Carotene – 4.8

Both of these and as it is for most vegetable also contains minerals in some measures as we can see for Spinach below:

Spinach (mg/100 g fresh weight) – Mineral contents:

K-Potassium – 554 good for lowering blood pressure if that is the focus;

Na – Sodium – 69 – good for increasing blood pressure

Ca- Calcium – 60

Mg- Magnesium – 117;

Fe- Iron- 3.8;

Mn- Manganese-0.6;

Co – Cobalt - 0.002

Cu – Copper – 0.1;

Zn – Zinc – 0.6;

P – Phosphorous – 46;

Cl- Chloride – 54

F- Fluorine – 0.08;

I – Iodine – 0.012

Needless to say, we got the point. A combination of one or two ingredients in a smoothie recipe can go a very long way in providing the required food intake, creating a fill sensation and help with weight correction. For the most part and best results these listed recipes are provided with no sugar added. Some nutritional benefits of some not so common ingredients have been added.

## Cacao Powder

Cacao power is used to make chocolates and some form of energy bars we enjoy so much. Wonder no more. This incredibly very nutritious ingredient packs a whopper when it comes to Recommended Dietary Allowance, RDA. It is also beneficial for improving blood flow and reducing blood pressure to mention a few.

For Example, according to Nutrition Advance (2) Cacao power contains:

- Manganese: 192% RDA

- Copper: 189% RDA

- Magnesium: 125% RDA

- Iron: 77% RDA

- Phosphorus: 73% RDA

Now we can see how overly beneficial this ingredient is. As a result, and for our own sake and what we want to achieve a small amount - a spoon or two - is recommended.

## Yogurt

According to (1) yogurt helps in lowering the risk of cardiovascular diseases. If It is fortified with probiotics the benefits even go further. For smoothies this is great. (9) even goes further to assert in a test on the health of children, that "significantly reduced days of fever, and an improved social and school functioning" Who knew?

## Avocado

If you must know Avocado is a fruit, but it is usually easily taken for a vegetable as used in salads and so on. It is nutrient laden, to the level that can be compared to that of Olive oil. Rich in Vitamins K, E, C, Copper and potassium. (12).

## Blackberries or berries in general

These are the most common ingredients we use in smoothies. They are very good for us and very healthy. Full of vitamins and minerals (6, 7,). Just make sure organic variants are used. In a randomised test it is asserted that Blueberries my help lower inflammation, blood pressure and oxidative stress (5).

## Tree Nuts

Tree nuts in general are favoured here as they are generally known for their beneficial properties. They are packed with minerals, like copper, manganese and vitamins like B1. They are also very good for lowering inflammation in the body (3).

## Milk

Milk have been very controversial in recent years due to the calcium content it may or may not contain. However totally discarding it is not recommended as some value is still been provided regardless of the benefits is still provides. Studies conducted by the National research council, (13), whole milk (only) may be beneficial for lowering risk of diabetes. Milk also contains apart from Calcium, Vitamin B, D, Protein and Phosphorus (8).

## Honey

Honey has been around for a very long time. It warms from the inside and as a sweetener a better choice that refined sugar for smoothies. Contains 100% Carbs, 0% fat and 0% protein (14). Depending on where your choice of honey coms from it mat contain different varieties on minerals and vitamins. It is recommended to use natural organic sources.

Banana a widely know fruit around the world. It is one of those ingredients that is very often used in smoothies, for the taste, basically as a substitution for sugar – this is recommended – and as a source of fiber. Banana also contains high levels of minerals like Potassium and vitamins

# Now to the Races, so To Say

1. Peach Walnut Cranberry Smoothie

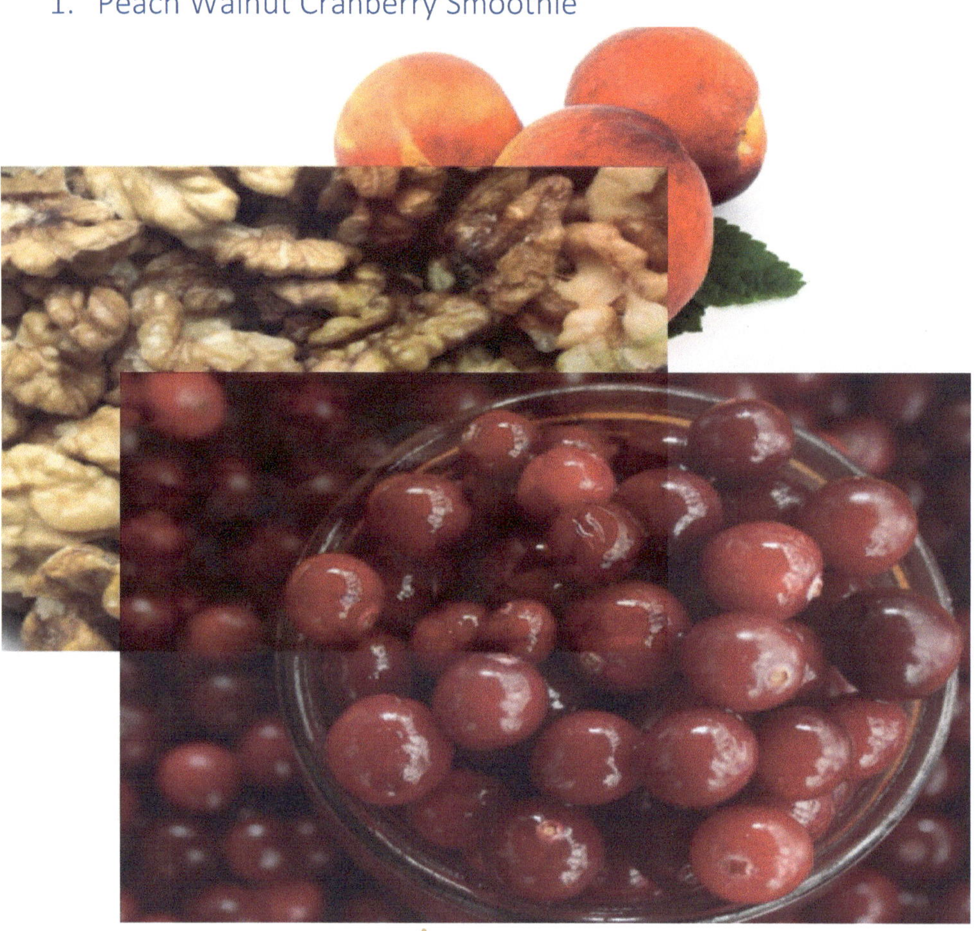

*Peach-Walnut-Cranberry*

Ingredients:

Half a fresh peach, cut into chunks

4 walnuts

1 cup plain yogurt

1 teaspoon vanilla extract

1 cup water or soymilk

## 2. Spinach Blueberry Oatmeal Avocado Smoothie

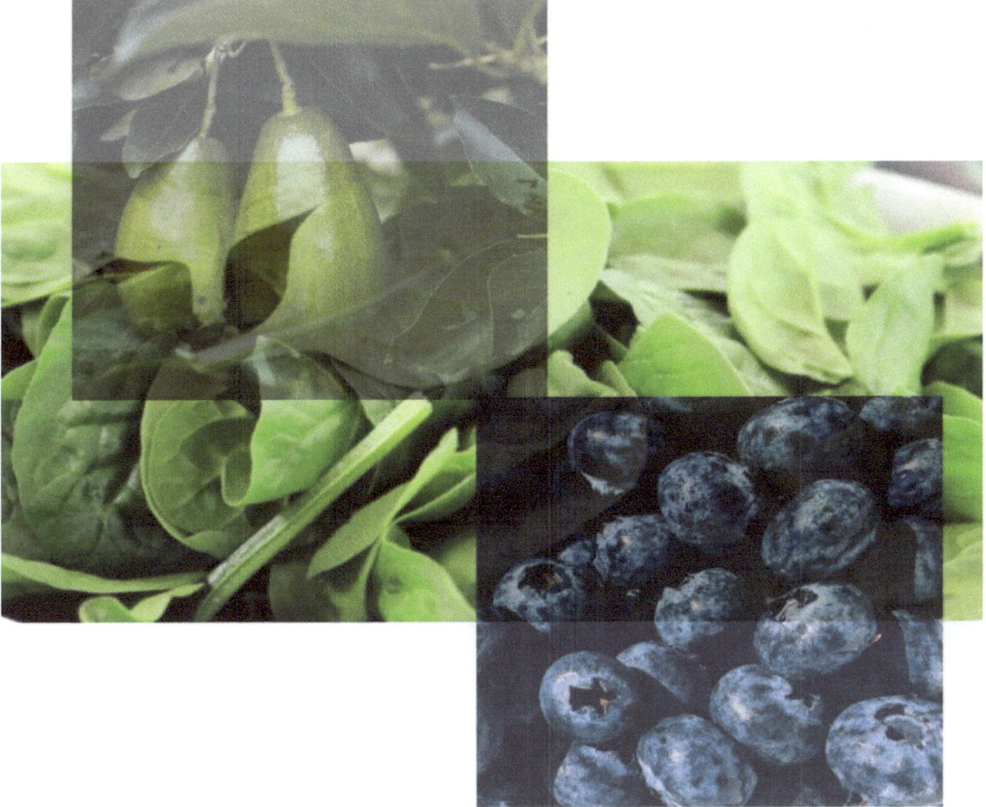

*Spinach-Blueberry-Avocado*

Ingredients:

1 Tbs. sunflower seeds

2 Tablespoons raw oats

1 cup fresh or frozen blueberries

1/2 cup frozen spinach

Half an avocado, cut into chunks

1 cup plain yogurt

water, milk or soymilk

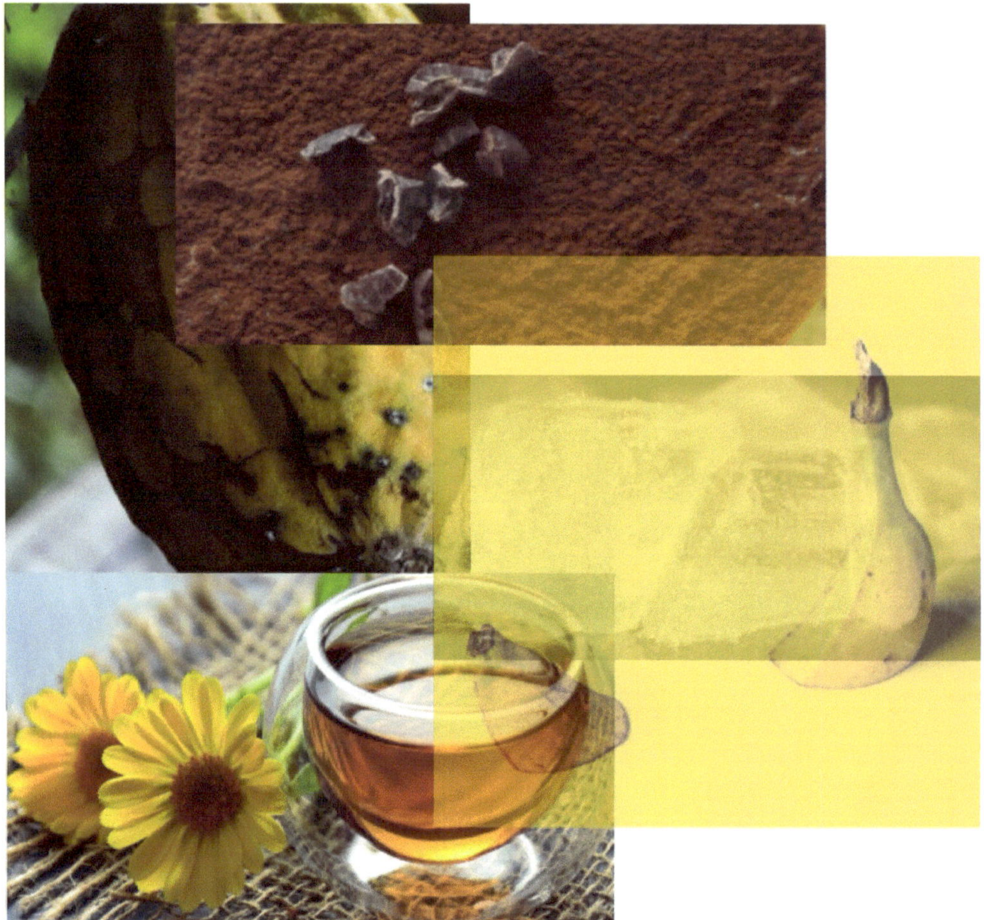

*Cocoa-Honey-Banana-Honey*

Ingredients:

1Tablespoon unsweetened cocoa powder

1 Tablespoon honey

1 banana

ice cubes

1 cup yogurt

water

This one here will surprise you wonderfully. We all know how Kale tastes like on its own. Fortified with vitamins and minerals no wonder it is recommended by nutritionist as one of the best nutritious herbs.

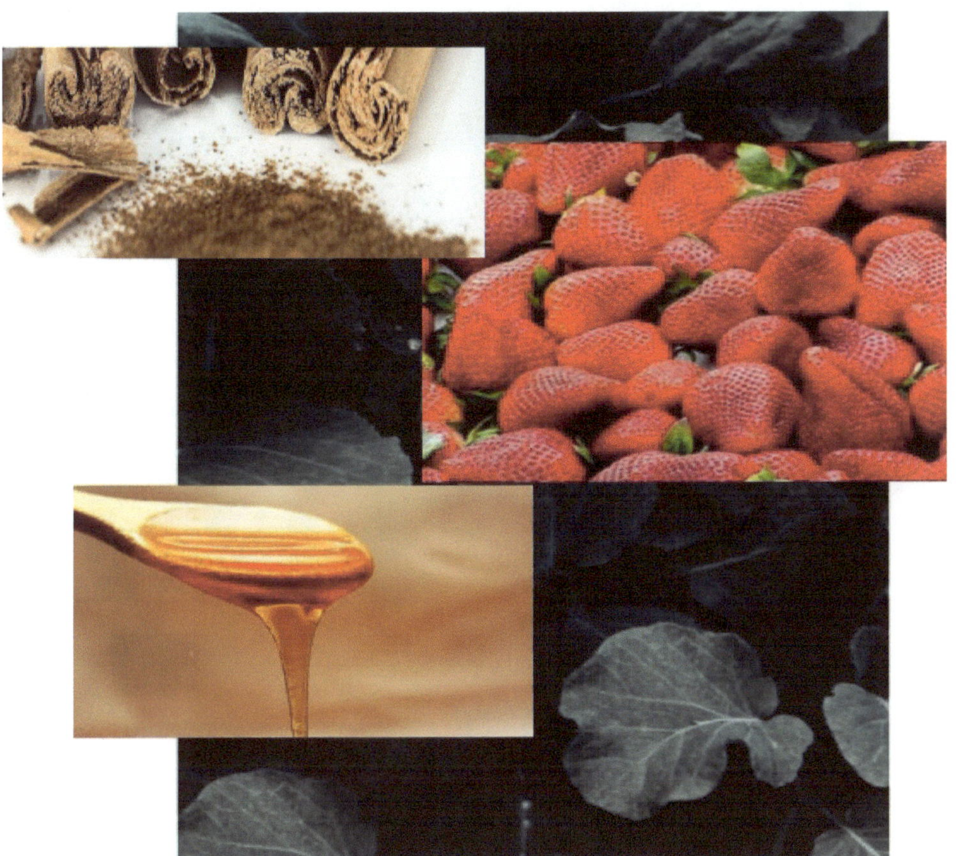

*Kale-Cinnamon-Honey-Strawberry*

Ingredients:

1 cup of frozen Strawberries

1/2 cup of fresh or frozen Kale

1 cup of plain Yogurt

1 Tablespoon of Honey

A Dash of Cinnamon

Add water or Soymilk

The resulting smoothie from this combination will look like nothing you have ever seen before.

## 5.  Raspberry Banana Pecan Smoothie

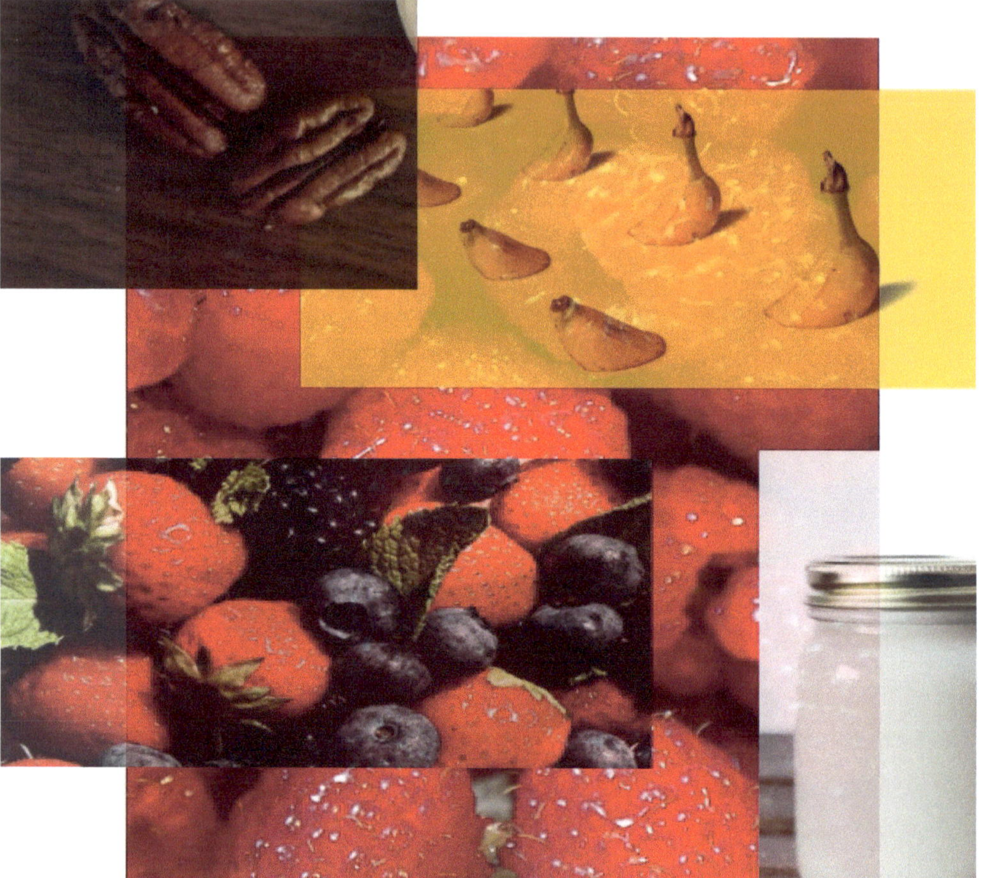

*Rapsberry-Bannana Smoothie*

Ingredients:

1/2 cup frozen raspberries

1/2 banana

4 pecans

1 cup yogurt

sprinkle of nutmeg

## 6.  Berry Blast Smoothie

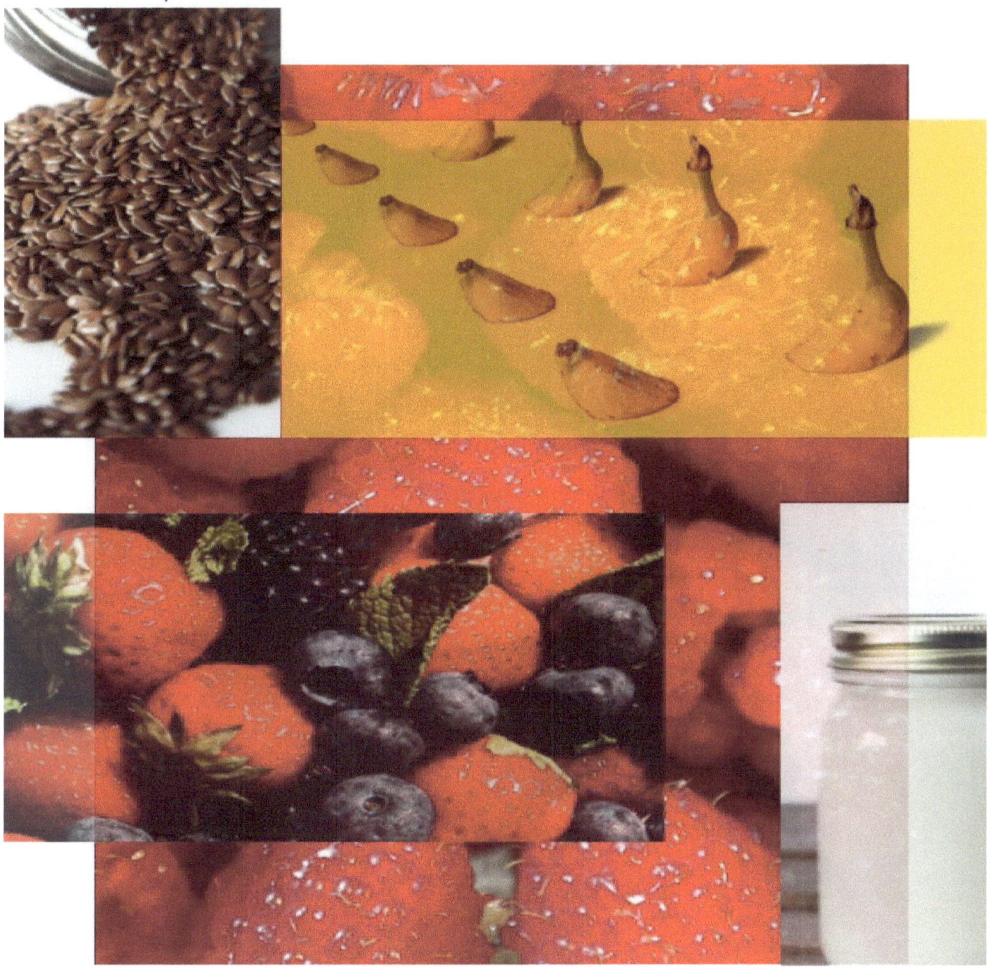

*Flaxseed-Berries-Banana*

Ingredients:

1 teaspoon Flaxseed

1 cup fresh or frozen mixed berries such as Strawberries, Blueberries, Raspberries

1 cup plain Yogurt

1 teaspoon Vanilla Extract

Add Water or Soymilk

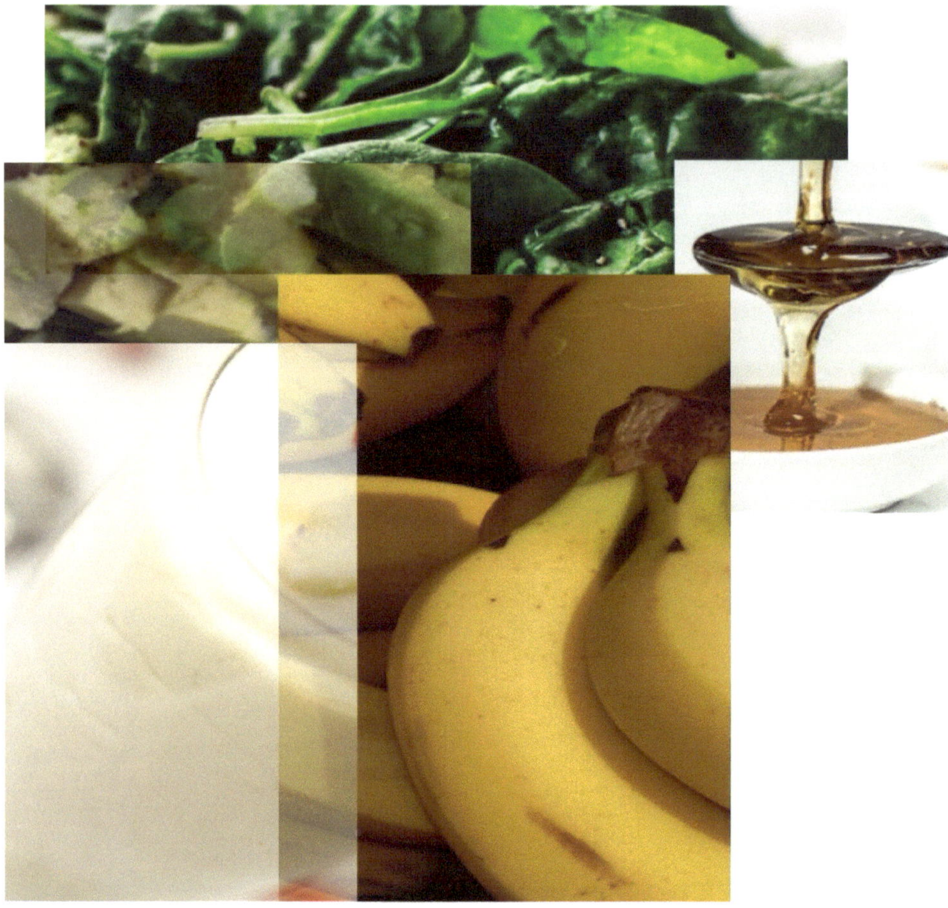

*Flaxseed-Berries-Banana*

Ingredients:

1/2 avocado, cut in chunks

1/2 cup frozen spinach

1 Tbs. honey

1/2 banana

1 cup plain yogurt

# Conclusion

In conclusion it is encouraged to experiment with different combinations as we desire. These are a just select few of what is possible. In time, more will be added in time. It is envisaged that you will love these as past experiences have shown. Please recommend as seen appropriate to friends and family members. To continue to provide well studied materials to and be better at it please let us know what you think about this publication and what you have tried and how it is working for you. Afterall, living healthy is a must to all and it is very simple and affordable to do.

Nutrition in itself as defines as the scientific interpretations of nutrients and related substances to promote health to maintain healthy living in all aspects of human and animals' lives from intake to excretion. It is very broad science and it is comforting that the world have started taking notice of this. Please remember that for the sake of this book it is all about food-type combinations for the best results. It is hoped that you will enjoy it. Buy it for yourself and family, lend it, share It, and buy it as a perfect gift for anyone.

# References


1.  Wu, L., & Sun, D. (2017). Consumption of Yogurt and the Incident Risk of Cardiovascular Disease: A Meta-Analysis of Nine Cohort Studies. *Nutrients*, *9*(3), 315. doi:10.3390/nu9030315

2.  Magrone, T., Russo, M. A., & Jirillo, E. (2017). Cocoa and Dark Chocolate Polyphenols: From Biology to Clinical Applications. *Frontiers in immunology*, *8*, 677. doi:10.3389/fimmu.2017.00677

3.  Liana C Del Gobbo, Michael C Falk, Robin Feldman, Kara Lewis, Dariush Mozaffarian, Effects of tree nuts on blood lipids, apolipoproteins, and blood pressure: systematic review, meta-analysis, and dose-response of 61 controlled intervention trials, *The American Journal of Clinical Nutrition*, Volume 102, Issue 6, December 2015, Pages 1347–1356, https://doi.org/10.3945/ajcn.115.110965

4.  Deirdre K Banel, Frank B Hu, Effects of walnut consumption on blood lipids and other cardiovascular risk factors: a meta-analysis and systematic review, *The American Journal of Clinical Nutrition*, Volume 90, Issue 1, July 2009, Pages 56–63, https://doi.org/10.3945/ajcn.2009.27457

5.  Aghababaee, S. K., Vafa, M., Shidfar, F., Tahavorgar, A., Gohari, M., Katebi, D., & Mohammadi, V. (2015). Effects of blackberry (Morus nigra L.) consumption on serum concentration of lipoproteins, apo A-I, apo B, and high-sensitivity-C-reactive protein and blood pressure in dyslipidemic patients. *Journal of research in medical sciences: the official journal of Isfahan University of Medical Sciences*, *20*(7), 684–691. doi:10.4103/1735-1995.166227

6.  Strawberries, raw Nutrition Facts & Calories. Self Nutrition Data. Reviewed on October 12, 2019 from: https://nutritiondata.self.com/facts/fruits-and-fruit-juices/2064/2

7.  Blueberries, raw Nutrition Facts & Calories. Self Nutrition Data. Reviewed on October 12, 2019 from: https://nutritiondata.self.com/facts/fruits-and-fruit-juices/1851/2

8.  National Research Council (US) Committee on Diet and Health. Diet and Health: Implications for Reducing Chronic Disease Risk. Washington (DC): National Academies Press (US); 1989. 11, Fat-Soluble Vitamins. Available from: https://www.ncbi.nlm.nih.gov/books/NBK218749/

9.  A systematic review of the effect of yogurt consumption on chronic diseases risk markers in adults. Audrée-Anne Dumas, Annie Lapointe, Marilyn Dugrenier, Véronique Provencher, Benoît Lamarche, Sophie Desroches Eur J Nutr. 2016 Nov 2 Published online 2016 Nov 2. doi: 10.1007/s00394-016-1341-7

10. Magrone, T., Russo, M. A., & Jirillo, E. (2017). Cocoa and Dark Chocolate Polyphenols: From Biology to Clinical Applications. *Frontiers in immunology*, *8*, 677. doi:10.3389/fimmu.2017.00677

11. Belitz, Hans-Dieter & Grosch, Werner & Schieberle, Peter. (2008). Vegetables and Vegetable Products. 10.1007/978-3-540-69934-7_18.

12. Avocados, raw, all commercial varieties Nutrition Facts & Calories. Self Nutrition Data. Reviewed on October 13, 2019 from: https://nutritiondata.self.com/facts/fruits-and-fruit-juices/1843/2

13. Milk, whole, 3.25% milkfat Nutrition Facts & Calories. Self Nutrition Data. Reviewed and from: https://nutritiondata.self.com/facts/dairy-and-egg-products/69/2

14. Honey Nutrition Facts & Calories. Self Nutrition Data. Reviewed on October 13, 2019 from: https://nutritiondata.self.com/facts/sweets/5568/2

15. 4 BIG Health Benefits of 12 Hour Intermittent Fasting. Clean Cuisine. Reviewed on October 13, 2019 from: https://cleancuisine.com/12-hour-intermittent-fasting/